WALL PILATES FOR BEGINNERS

Mary Dixon

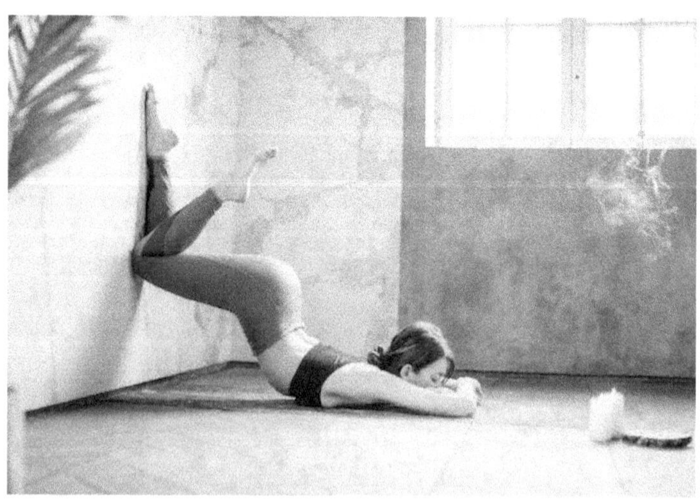

TABLE OF CONTENT

CHAPTER ONE

Introduction to Wall Pilates

Pilates is a fitness method that has gained immense popularity for its ability to improve strength, flexibility, and overall well-being. It was developed by Joseph Pilates in the early 20th century and has since evolved into various forms and variations to cater to different fitness levels and needs. One such adaptation that has gained prominence in recent years is "Wall Pilates."

Wall Pilates combines the principles of traditional Pilates with the support of a wall, making it a versatile and accessible exercise modality suitable for individuals of all fitness levels, including beginners.

This fusion allows participants to experience the core tenets of Pilates while utilizing the stability and resistance provided by a vertical surface. In this introduction, we will delve into the essence of Wall Pilates, its origins, benefits, and the reasons why it has become a sought-after fitness regimen for individuals seeking improved posture, core strength, and flexibility.

The Foundation of Pilates

To understand Wall Pilates, it is essential to first grasp the core principles of Pilates. Joseph Pilates, the founder of this method, believed that physical and mental health are intertwined and can be improved through a disciplined and controlled approach to exercise. He developed a series of movements that emphasize core strength, proper alignment, breath control, and a mind-body connection. These principles remain at the heart of Wall Pilates.

What is Wall Pilates?

Wall Pilates, as the name suggests, incorporates a wall into traditional Pilates exercises. It provides a stable support system that allows participants to work on their alignment, engage specific muscle groups, and maintain balance during movements. The wall is used as both a guide and a resistance source, enabling individuals to gain a deeper understanding of their bodies and movements.

In Wall Pilates, participants use the wall to perform exercises such as squats, leg lifts, stretches, and more. The wall acts as a constant reference point, promoting proper form and alignment.

This approach helps individuals to focus on the targeted muscle groups, making the exercises more effective.

Benefits of Wall Pilates

Wall Pilates offers a wide range of benefits that can enhance both physical and mental well-being. Some of the key advantages of Wall Pilates include:

1. Improved Posture: Wall Pilates emphasizes correct spinal alignment, which can help alleviate issues related to poor posture. By maintaining proper posture during exercises, participants can carry these principles into their daily lives.

2. Core Strength: A strong core is crucial for overall physical fitness and well-being. Wall Pilates targets the core muscles, including the abdominal and lower back muscles, helping individuals build a solid foundation of strength.

3. Flexibility: The controlled and deliberate movements of Wall Pilates help improve flexibility, making it an ideal choice for those seeking enhanced range of motion and reduced muscle tightness.

4. Body Awareness: Wall Pilates places a strong emphasis on the mind-body connection. By focusing on each movement and maintaining a mindful approach, participants can develop a heightened awareness of their bodies.

5. Injury Prevention: The controlled and low-impact nature of Wall Pilates makes it an excellent choice for injury prevention and rehabilitation. It is gentle on the joints, making it accessible to individuals of varying fitness levels and ages.

6. Stress Reduction: Pilates, including Wall Pilates, promotes relaxation and stress reduction. The deep breathing and focus required during the exercises can have a calming effect on the mind and body.

Wall Pilates is not just about physical fitness but also about cultivating a sense of balance and harmony within oneself. It offers a holistic approach to health and wellness that can be adapted to individual needs and goals.

Whether you are a beginner looking for an entry point into the world of Pilates or an experienced practitioner seeking a fresh perspective, Wall Pilates has something to offer.

The Basics of Pilates

Pilates is a unique and comprehensive fitness method that focuses on the development of core strength, flexibility, balance, and overall body awareness.

Created by Joseph Pilates in the early 20th century, it has since gained widespread popularity for its holistic approach to physical fitness and well-being. The core principles of Pilates, which form the foundation of the practice, are essential to understanding this exercise system.

Core Principles of Pilates:

1. Concentration: Pilates places a strong emphasis on the mind-body connection. Concentration is a key principle, encouraging individuals to focus on the precise execution of each movement. By paying close attention to the quality of movement, participants can enhance their body awareness and achieve optimal results.

2. Control: Control in Pilates refers to the precise and deliberate execution of exercises. It's not about quantity but quality. Movements are performed with a sense of grace and fluidity, with the goal of developing control over the body's movements and alignment.

3. Centering: The center of the body, often referred to as the "powerhouse," is pivotal in Pilates. It encompasses the muscles of the abdomen, lower back, pelvis, and buttocks. Strengthening this area is fundamental to Pilates, as it provides stability and support for all movements.

4. Precision: Pilates is all about precision in movement. It encourages practitioners to perform exercises with exactness, paying attention to proper alignment, and avoiding unnecessary strain or tension. Precision ensures that the right muscles are targeted and engaged.

5. Breath: Proper breathing is crucial in Pilates. It is coordinated with movement, and the emphasis is on deep, diaphragmatic breathing. Breath control enhances oxygenation of the body, improves focus, and helps to release tension.

6. Flow: The smooth and continuous flow of movements is a hallmark of Pilates. Exercises are designed to flow seamlessly from one to the next, promoting a sense of harmony and balance in the body. Flow creates a dynamic and engaging practice.

7. Alignment: Correct alignment is vital in Pilates to prevent strain and injury. It is essential to maintain a neutral spine and pelvis while performing exercises. The focus on alignment promotes good posture and overall body awareness.

Equipment and Mat-Based Pilates

Pilates can be practiced using specialized equipment such as the Reformer, Cadillac, and the Wunda Chair, which offer varying degrees of resistance and support. However, mat-based Pilates is equally effective and accessible to most individuals.

Mat-based Pilates uses your body weight and gravity as resistance, and it can be done in the comfort of your own home or in a class setting with minimal equipment.

Who Can Benefit from Pilates?

Pilates is suitable for individuals of all ages and fitness levels. Whether you're a beginner looking to improve your overall well-being or an athlete seeking to enhance your performance, Pilates can be adapted to your specific needs and goals. It is especially beneficial for those looking to:

- Strengthen the core muscles.

- Improve posture and alignment.

- Increase flexibility and range of motion.

- Enhance overall body strength.

- Rehabilitate from injuries or manage chronic conditions.

- Develop a balanced and harmonious body.

Pilates is more than just a workout; it is a holistic approach to physical fitness and well-being.

By understanding and applying the core principles of Pilates and choosing the appropriate approach, whether mat-based or equipment-based, individuals can embark on a journey of self-discovery, improved strength, and enhanced overall health.

Whether you are a beginner or an experienced practitioner, Pilates has something valuable to offer to support your fitness and wellness goals.

What is Wall Pilates?

Wall Pilates is a specialized variation of the traditional Pilates method that incorporates the use of a wall as a support and resistance tool during exercise.

This innovative approach combines the fundamental principles of Pilates with the added benefit of a vertical surface, allowing practitioners to perform a wide range of movements that emphasize core strength, flexibility, balance, and overall body awareness.

The key features of Wall Pilates include:

1. Wall as a Support: In Wall Pilates, the wall serves as a stable and supportive structure. It provides a reference point for proper alignment, which is crucial in Pilates, and allows individuals to maintain their balance during exercises. The wall offers a sense of security, making it an ideal choice for beginners or those who may struggle with balance issues.

2. Alignment and Form: Wall Pilates places a strong emphasis on correct body alignment. Practitioners can use the wall to guide them in maintaining the right posture throughout each exercise, preventing unnecessary strain and promoting optimal muscle engagement.

3. Resistance and Intensity: The wall also acts as a resistance source, enabling individuals to perform exercises that engage various muscle groups while using the wall's support.

This added resistance can increase the intensity of the movements, making Wall Pilates effective for strength building.

4. Versatility: Wall Pilates can be adapted to accommodate different fitness levels and goals. It offers a wide range of exercises, from basic stretches to more advanced movements, allowing individuals to progressively challenge themselves as they become more proficient.

5. Balance and Stability: Wall Pilates helps develop core strength, which is essential for stability and balance. By utilizing the wall for support and resistance, practitioners can enhance their balance and coordination, making it a valuable addition to rehabilitation programs and sports-specific training.

6. Mind-Body Connection: Similar to traditional Pilates, Wall Pilates promotes the mind-body connection. Practitioners are encouraged to focus on their breath, engage their core, and maintain concentration during each movement, fostering a sense of mindfulness and inner awareness.

7. Low Impact: Wall Pilates is a low-impact exercise method, making it suitable for individuals with joint issues or those who prefer a gentle and safe approach to fitness.

The exercises in Wall Pilates can range from wall squats and leg lifts to wall angels, roll downs, leg circles, and bridging.

These movements target various muscle groups, including the core, legs, arms, and back, providing a full-body workout that emphasizes strength, flexibility, and posture improvement.

Wall Pilates can be practiced in a variety of settings, including fitness studios, rehabilitation centers, and even in the comfort of your own home with minimal equipment. It is adaptable to individual needs and fitness levels, making it an excellent choice for both beginners and experienced

Pilates enthusiasts who are looking for a fresh and effective approach to their fitness routine. Whether you're seeking improved core strength, better posture, enhanced flexibility, or a comprehensive mind-body workout, Wall Pilates offers a unique and versatile method to help you achieve your fitness and wellness goals.

Benefits of Wall Pilates

Wall Pilates offers a wide range of benefits for individuals of all fitness levels, making it a valuable addition to one's exercise routine. These benefits encompass physical, mental, and even rehabilitative aspects, making Wall Pilates a versatile and holistic approach to fitness. Here are some of the key advantages of practicing Wall Pilates:

1. Improved Posture: Wall Pilates places a strong emphasis on correct body alignment. By using the wall as a reference point, participants can develop better posture, both during exercise and in their everyday lives. This is particularly beneficial for individuals who spend long hours sitting at desks or engaging in activities that can lead to poor posture.

2. Core Strength: Wall Pilates targets the core muscles, including the abdominals, lower back, and pelvic muscles. Strengthening the core is essential for overall body stability and helps to prevent and alleviate back pain and discomfort.

3. Flexibility: The controlled and deliberate movements in Wall Pilates help improve flexibility. Over time, participants can experience increased range of motion, reduced muscle tightness, and enhanced mobility, which is especially beneficial for those looking to maintain or regain flexibility as they age.

4. Body Awareness: Wall Pilates promotes mindfulness and body awareness. By focusing on each movement and maintaining a mindful approach, participants can develop a heightened sense of their bodies, how they move, and where they may have imbalances or weaknesses.

5. Low Impact: Wall Pilates is a low-impact exercise method, making it suitable for individuals of various fitness levels and ages. It is gentle on the joints, making it a safer option for those with joint issues or who are recovering from injuries.

6. Strength and Endurance: Wall Pilates can be adapted to offer progressive strength and endurance challenges. As you become more proficient, you can increase the intensity of the exercises to build overall body strength.

7. Stress Reduction: The deep breathing and focus required during Wall Pilates exercises can have a calming effect on the mind and body. It can help reduce stress and promote relaxation.

8. Injury Prevention and Rehabilitation: Wall Pilates can be used for injury prevention and rehabilitation. The controlled movements and focus on alignment make it an excellent choice for those looking to recover from injuries or manage chronic conditions.

9. Versatility: Wall Pilates offers a wide variety of exercises that can be tailored to individual needs and goals. Whether you are looking to tone specific muscle groups, improve your balance, or simply enhance your overall well-being, Wall Pilates can be adapted to your unique requirements.

10. Mind-Body Connection: Like traditional Pilates, Wall Pilates encourages the development of a strong mind-body connection. Practitioners learn to focus on their breath, engage their core, and maintain concentration during each movement, which can lead to a greater sense of inner awareness and mindfulness.

11. Balance and Coordination: The stability provided by the wall in Wall Pilates exercises helps individuals develop better balance and coordination. This can be particularly beneficial for athletes and those seeking to improve their balance and functional fitness.

Who Can Benefit from Wall Pilates?

Wall Pilates is a versatile and accessible exercise method that offers a wide range of benefits and can be adapted to suit various fitness levels and individual needs. As such, a broad spectrum of individuals can benefit from Wall Pilates. Here are some of the groups of people who can benefit from Wall Pilates:

1. Beginners: Wall Pilates is an excellent choice for beginners who are new to Pilates or fitness in general. The wall provides additional support, making it easier for novices to learn and execute exercises with proper form and alignment.

2. Intermediate and Advanced Practitioners: Even experienced Pilates practitioners can benefit from Wall Pilates. It offers a new dimension to their practice by adding resistance and versatility to their routine, allowing them to further challenge their strength, flexibility, and balance.

3. Athletes: Athletes from various sports can integrate Wall Pilates into their training routines. It helps improve core strength, flexibility, and balance, which are essential for enhancing athletic performance and preventing injuries.

4. Seniors: Wall Pilates is well-suited for seniors as it is gentle on the joints and can help maintain or improve flexibility, balance, and muscle strength, promoting overall functional fitness and quality of life.

5. Individuals with Limited Mobility: Wall Pilates can be adapted to accommodate individuals with limited mobility. The support of the wall makes it possible for those with physical challenges to engage in a beneficial exercise routine.

6. Individuals with Back Pain: People dealing with back pain or discomfort may find relief through Wall Pilates. The focus on core strength and proper alignment can help alleviate back issues and prevent further discomfort.

7. Those Seeking Rehabilitation: Wall Pilates can be a valuable addition to rehabilitation programs. The controlled and low-impact nature of the exercises is ideal for those recovering from injuries or surgeries.

8. Office Workers: Individuals who spend long hours sitting at a desk or working on computers can benefit from Wall Pilates to counteract the effects of poor posture and prolonged sitting, leading to improved posture and reduced back pain.

9. Pregnant Women: Wall Pilates can be adapted for pregnant women, helping them maintain core strength and flexibility during pregnancy while emphasizing safety and comfort.

10. Stress Reduction Seekers: The focus on deep breathing and mindfulness in Wall Pilates can help individuals manage stress and promote relaxation.

11. Fitness Enthusiasts: Those who are already active and enjoy other forms of exercise can use Wall Pilates to complement their existing fitness routines, targeting specific muscle groups and adding variety to their workouts.

12. Individuals with Postural Issues: Wall Pilates is particularly beneficial for those with postural issues, as it places a strong emphasis on alignment and can help individuals develop better posture over time.

It's important to note that Wall Pilates is highly adaptable and can be customized to suit individual needs and goals. Whether you're looking to improve core strength, flexibility, balance, or overall well-being, Wall Pilates offers a versatile approach to fitness that can benefit a diverse range of individuals.

As with any new exercise program, it's recommended to consult with a healthcare professional or qualified instructor to ensure that Wall Pilates is safe and appropriate for your specific circumstances.

Safety Precautions and Guidelines

Safety is paramount when engaging in any form of physical activity, including Wall Pilates. While Wall Pilates is generally safe and suitable for a wide range of individuals, it's essential to follow safety precautions and guidelines to minimize the risk of injury and ensure a positive and effective experience. Here are some important safety precautions and guidelines for practicing Wall Pilates:

1. Consult with a Healthcare Professional: Before beginning any exercise program, it's advisable to consult with a healthcare professional or a qualified Pilates instructor, especially if you have any pre-existing medical conditions, injuries, or concerns.

2. Choose a Qualified Instructor: If you're new to Wall Pilates, consider working with a certified and experienced

Pilates instructor. They can provide guidance, ensure proper form, and tailor exercises to your specific needs and abilities.

3. Warm-Up: Always begin your Wall Pilates session with a gentle warm-up to prepare your body for exercise. Warm-up exercises can include light stretching, deep breathing, and gentle mobility movements.

4. Proper Attire: Wear comfortable, breathable clothing that allows for a full range of motion. Avoid clothing that is too loose, as it may obstruct your view of your body's alignment during exercises.

5. Use a Suitable Wall: Ensure that the wall you use for Wall Pilates is stable, free from obstacles, and has a clean, dry surface. Avoid using walls with rough or abrasive textures that could cause skin irritation.

6. Footwear: In most Wall Pilates exercises, you'll perform movements barefoot or in grip socks. These provide better stability and control, allowing you to feel the wall's support and resistance more effectively.

7. Focus on Alignment: Pay close attention to proper body alignment during each exercise. The wall is your reference point for alignment, so use it to maintain good posture and avoid straining muscles or joints.

8. Breath Control: Coordinate your breath with your movements. Inhale through your nose to prepare, and exhale through your mouth to execute the movement. Breathing helps with concentration, control, and relaxation.

9. Progress Gradually: Start with basic Wall Pilates exercises, and as you become more comfortable and proficient, gradually progress to more advanced movements. Don't push yourself too hard too quickly.

10. Avoid Overexertion: Listen to your body and avoid overexertion. If you experience pain, discomfort, or dizziness during a Wall Pilates exercise, stop immediately and consult a healthcare professional if necessary.

11. Stay Hydrated: Drink plenty of water before, during, and after your Wall Pilates session to stay hydrated. Dehydration can affect your performance and overall well-being.

12. Rest and Recovery: Allow your body to rest and recover between Wall Pilates sessions. Consistency is key, but it's equally important to avoid overtraining.

13. Progress Tracking: Keep a record of your progress and performance. Tracking your achievements can help you set and achieve fitness goals while ensuring you're making safe and gradual improvements.

14. Modify for Individual Needs: Wall Pilates exercises can be modified to accommodate individual abilities and limitations. Always choose exercises and variations that suit your specific needs and goals.

15. Discontinue if Necessary: If you experience pain or discomfort that persists, consult a healthcare professional and consider modifying or discontinuing specific exercises as needed.

By following these safety precautions and guidelines, you can enhance your Wall Pilates practice while minimizing the risk of injury. Safety and proper technique are essential for a successful and enjoyable Wall Pilates experience.

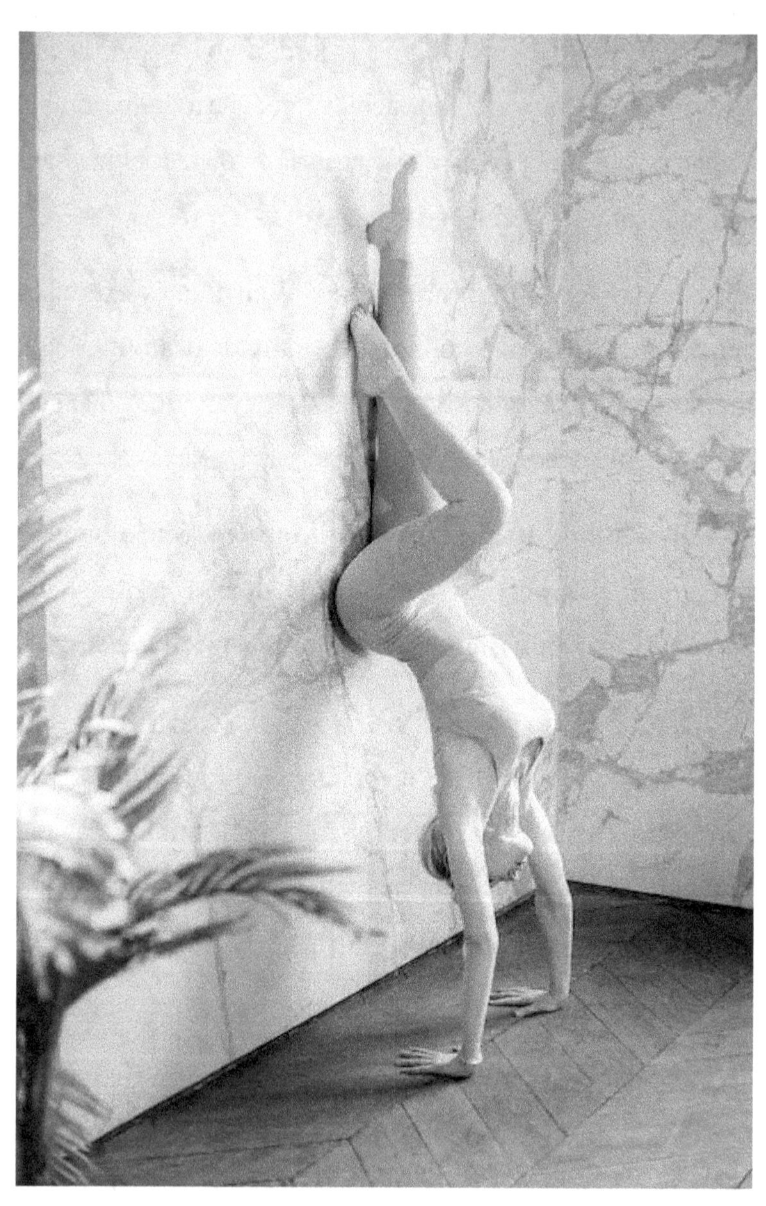

CHAPTER TWO

Getting Started with Wall Pilates

Wall Pilates, a unique and innovative variation of the traditional Pilates method, offers a dynamic approach to building strength, improving balance, and enhancing flexibility. This introductory guide will help you embark on your Wall Pilates journey, exploring the fundamental principles, equipment, and techniques that will empower you to experience the benefits of this versatile exercise system.

Embracing the Pilates Legacy

Joseph Pilates, the visionary creator of the Pilates method, once said, "Physical fitness is the first requisite of happiness." His dedication to the mind-body connection and the importance of controlled, deliberate movement laid the foundation for what we know today as Pilates. Wall Pilates, as a modern extension of this legacy, preserves these core principles while introducing the support and resistance of a wall to amplify the experience.

The Basics of Pilates

Before diving into Wall Pilates, it's essential to understand the essence of Pilates itself. Pilates is not just a workout; it is a holistic approach to physical fitness and well-being. At its core, Pilates emphasizes several key principles:

- Concentration: Focused attention on precise execution of movements.
- Control: Deliberate and smooth movements, avoiding unnecessary tension.
- Centering: Activation of the body's core muscles for stability and strength.
- Precision: Exact execution of exercises, emphasizing proper alignment.
- Breath: Coordination of breath with movement for optimal oxygenation.
- Flow: Fluidity and continuity of movements to create a sense of harmony.

These principles transcend into Wall Pilates, where they combine with the wall's support and resistance, fostering a mindful and balanced approach to physical fitness.

The Wall as Your Ally

In Wall Pilates, the wall becomes your ally in every movement. It offers support, guidance, and resistance, creating a unique workout environment that is both challenging and empowering.

The wall provides stability and structure, allowing you to maintain alignment and balance as you execute exercises. It acts as your constant reference point, helping you understand your body's positioning and muscle engagement.

The Benefits of Wall Pilates

Wall Pilates offers a myriad of benefits, making it an appealing choice for individuals of various fitness levels and backgrounds. Here are some of the advantages you can expect from practicing Wall Pilates:

1. Improved Posture: Wall Pilates places a strong emphasis on correct alignment, which can help alleviate issues related to poor posture.

2. Core Strength: A strong core is crucial for overall physical fitness and well-being. Wall Pilates targets the core muscles, helping you build a solid foundation of strength.

3. Flexibility: The controlled and deliberate movements of Wall Pilates help improve flexibility, making it an ideal choice for those seeking enhanced range of motion and reduced muscle tightness.

4. Body Awareness: Wall Pilates promotes body awareness and mindfulness, helping you connect with your body and movements on a deeper level.

5. Balance and Stability: The wall's support enhances balance and stability, making it an excellent choice for those looking to improve their coordination and functional fitness.

6. Low-Impact: Wall Pilates is gentle on the joints, making it accessible to individuals of varying fitness levels and ages.

Your Journey Begins

Now that you've gained a foundational understanding of Wall Pilates and its principles, you're ready to start your journey. In the chapters that follow, we will delve into the practical aspects of Wall Pilates, including setting up your space, understanding essential equipment, and mastering warm-up exercises to prepare your body for the transformative experience that Wall Pilates offers.

Wall Pilates is not just a workout; it's a pathway to enhanced well-being, strength, and balance. Whether you're a beginner or an experienced practitioner looking for a fresh perspective, Wall Pilates has something to offer. The wall becomes your partner in this journey, guiding you towards a healthier, more harmonious relationship with your body and movement. It's time to step up to the wall, embrace the power of Wall Pilates, and unlock your full potential in the world of mindful fitness.

Setting up Your Space

Creating an ideal space for your Wall Pilates practice is an essential step in ensuring a safe and effective workout experience. Your environment plays a significant role in promoting focus, comfort, and motivation during your sessions. In this chapter, we'll explore the key considerations for setting up your Wall Pilates space to maximize the benefits of this unique exercise method.

Finding the Right Location

Selecting the right location for your Wall Pilates practice is the first and most crucial step in setting up your space. Here are some factors to consider:

1. Open Space: Choose an area with enough open space to accommodate your Wall Pilates movements comfortably. You should be able to fully extend your arms and legs without encountering obstacles.

2. Clean and Tidy: Ensure that your practice area is clean and free from clutter. A tidy environment can contribute to a calm and focused mindset.

3. Good Lighting: Natural light is ideal, as it can help boost your mood and energy levels. If natural light is not available, opt for well-lit artificial lighting to create a welcoming atmosphere.

4. Ventilation: Proper ventilation is essential to maintain a comfortable temperature during your workouts. Make sure the room is well-ventilated, especially if you plan to break a sweat.

5. Privacy: Choose a space where you feel comfortable and free from distractions. The ability to concentrate without interruptions is essential for a successful practice.

6. Mirror: While not a necessity, having a full-length mirror in your practice area can be beneficial. It allows you to check your form and alignment during exercises, promoting better posture and technique.

Flooring and Surface

The type of flooring or surface in your practice area is a critical consideration. Look for flooring options that provide cushioning and support to protect your joints and ensure a safe and comfortable practice. Here are some options:

1. Pilates Mat: A Pilates mat is an excellent choice for most Wall Pilates exercises. It provides a comfortable and supportive surface while offering grip to prevent slipping.

2. Carpet: A padded carpet can also serve as an adequate surface for Wall Pilates. Ensure it is clean, even, and free from irregularities that might affect balance and stability.

3. Wood or Hardwood Floor: If you're practicing Wall Pilates on a hardwood floor, consider using a Pilates mat or adding additional padding to protect your joints and provide extra cushioning.

4. Yoga Mat or Exercise Mat: If you're in a pinch and don't have a Pilates mat, a yoga mat or exercise mat can serve as a temporary solution. However, these may not provide the same level of support as a dedicated Pilates mat.

Wall Setup

The wall itself is a key element in Wall Pilates, and its setup is crucial for safety and effectiveness. Here's how to set up your wall for Wall Pilates:

1. Clear Wall Space: Ensure that the wall is free from obstructions, such as furniture, decor, or objects that might interfere with your movements.

2. Smooth and Clean Surface: The wall should have a smooth and clean surface to prevent skin irritation during exercises. Avoid walls with rough or abrasive textures.

3. Mounting Equipment: If you're using wall-mounted Pilates equipment, such as wall anchors or brackets, ensure they are securely installed by following the manufacturer's guidelines. These mounting points will be used to attach resistance bands or other equipment.

4. Sufficient Space: Ensure that the wall has enough space for you to extend your arms and legs fully during exercises without any restrictions.

Decor and Atmosphere

Personalize your Wall Pilates space to create a motivating and inviting atmosphere. This can enhance your overall experience and encourage regular practice:

1. Motivational Decor: Add elements that inspire you, such as posters, artwork, or motivational quotes that encourage you to stay committed to your practice.

2. Plant Life: Indoor plants can contribute to a calming and oxygen-rich environment. They can also improve air quality and create a pleasant atmosphere.

3. Music or Ambiance: Consider playing calming or energizing music that complements your practice. Alternatively, you can create a serene ambiance with soothing sounds or lighting.

4. Comfort: Ensure your practice area is comfortable by adding pillows, blankets, or cushions that can be used for support or relaxation during certain exercises.

By carefully considering the location, surface, wall setup, and overall atmosphere of your Wall Pilates space, you can create a welcoming and supportive environment that enhances your practice. A well-prepared space will help you focus on your exercises, maintain proper alignment, and fully reap the benefits of Wall Pilates.

Essential Equipment and Accessories

Wall Pilates incorporates unique equipment and accessories that are designed to enhance your practice, offering support, resistance, and versatility.

While it's possible to perform Wall Pilates exercises with minimal equipment, having the right tools can provide added benefits and variety to your workouts.

1. Pilates Mat:

A Pilates mat is an essential piece of equipment for Wall Pilates, providing a comfortable and supportive surface for your exercises. It offers cushioning for your joints and grip to prevent slipping, ensuring a safe and comfortable practice. Choose a mat that is thick enough to provide adequate padding.

2. Resistance Bands:

Resistance bands are versatile accessories that can be attached to the wall or other anchor points for added resistance during Wall Pilates exercises. They come in various levels of resistance, allowing you to tailor your workouts to your fitness level. Resistance bands are especially useful for enhancing strength and building muscle.

3. Yoga Straps:

Yoga straps, or stretching straps, can be used to assist with stretching and flexibility exercises. They allow you to deepen your stretches and improve your range of motion, making them a valuable addition to your Wall Pilates equipment.

4. Pilates Balls:

Pilates balls, also known as stability balls, can be incorporated into Wall Pilates exercises to challenge your balance and stability. They are often used for core-strengthening exercises and are available in various sizes to accommodate different fitness levels.

5. Pilates Magic Circle:

The Pilates Magic Circle is a flexible ring that can be used to add resistance to Wall Pilates exercises. It's particularly effective for targeting specific muscle groups, such as the inner and outer thighs, and can enhance the intensity of your workouts.

6. Grip Socks:

Grip socks have nonslip soles that provide added traction and stability during exercises. They are especially useful when performing movements on the wall, helping you maintain a firm grip and prevent slipping.

7. Wall-Mounted Equipment:

For a more advanced Wall Pilates setup, you can consider wall-mounted equipment such as wall anchors or brackets. These mounting points can be used to attach resistance bands, suspension trainers, or other Pilates accessories, expanding the range of exercises you can perform.

8. Mirror:

While not strictly an equipment item, having a full-length mirror in your practice space can be beneficial for Wall Pilates. It allows you to check your form and alignment during exercises, helping you maintain proper posture and technique.

9. Pilates Reformer (Optional):

Although not essential for beginners, a Pilates reformer is a specialized piece of equipment that can provide a comprehensive and challenging Wall Pilates experience. Reformer exercises are known for their versatility, offering both resistance and support.

10. Pilates Wall Charts:

Wall charts can serve as visual aids, displaying a variety of Wall Pilates exercises and proper form. They can be a helpful reference to ensure you're performing movements correctly.

The specific equipment and accessories you choose will depend on your fitness goals, budget, and the space you have available for your Wall Pilates practice.

You can start with the basics, such as a Pilates mat and resistance bands, and gradually expand your collection as you become more experienced and want to diversify your workouts. Remember to follow the instructions provided with your equipment and practice proper technique to ensure safe and effective Wall Pilates sessions.

Proper Attire for Wall Pilates

Choosing the right attire for Wall Pilates is essential for ensuring your comfort, safety, and the effectiveness of your workout. The ideal clothing and footwear should allow for a full range of motion, prevent slipping, and promote proper alignment during exercises. Here are some guidelines for selecting proper attire for your Wall Pilates sessions:

Clothing:

1. Comfortable and Form-Fitting: Opt for comfortable, form-fitting clothing that allows you to move freely without restriction. Loose or baggy clothing can interfere with your movements and make it challenging to maintain proper alignment.

2. Breathable Fabrics: Choose clothing made from breathable, moisture-wicking fabrics that help keep you cool and dry. Pilates sessions can be physically demanding, so clothing that wicks away sweat can enhance your overall comfort.

3. Layers: Layering can be practical, allowing you to adjust your clothing based on the temperature of your practice space. You can wear a lightweight top over a sports bra or tank top.

4. Avoid Jewelry: It's advisable to remove any jewelry that may get in the way or cause discomfort during exercises. This includes rings, bracelets, necklaces, or dangling earrings.

5. Avoid Zippers and Buttons: Clothing with zippers, buttons, or large embellishments can be uncomfortable when lying on your back or pressing against the wall. Look for seamless options to prevent irritation.

6. No Belted Pants: Avoid pants with belts, as they can dig into your skin and create pressure points when performing exercises, especially when lying on your back.

Footwear:

1. Barefoot or Grip Socks: Wall Pilates exercises are typically performed either barefoot or in grip socks with nonslip soles. Bare feet allow for better grip and tactile feedback during exercises. Grip socks provide traction and stability while protecting your feet.

2. Minimalist Shoes: If you prefer to wear shoes, opt for minimalist shoes with thin soles that allow for natural

movement. Avoid heavily cushioned or bulky shoes, as they can impede balance and stability.

Hair and Accessories:

1. Secure Hair: If you have long hair, it's a good idea to secure it in a bun, ponytail, or braids to prevent it from getting in your face and interfering with your movements.

2. Headbands: If you use headbands to keep hair off your face, choose ones that are snug but not too tight to avoid discomfort.

3. Minimal Accessories: Keep accessories to a minimum. While stud earrings and minimal jewelry are generally safe, avoid anything that may get caught or cause discomfort during exercises.

By following these guidelines, you can ensure that your attire enhances your Wall Pilates experience, allowing you to move freely, maintain proper alignment, and focus on the core principles of Pilates.

Comfort and safety are key when selecting the right clothing and footwear for your practice.

Warm-up Exercises

A proper warm-up is essential before beginning your Wall Pilates practice. Warming up helps prepare your body for exercise, increases blood flow to your muscles, and reduces the risk of injury. It also helps improve your flexibility and range of motion. Here are some effective warm-up exercises that you can incorporate into your Wall Pilates routine:

1. Neck Rolls:

- Stand with your feet hip-width apart.
- Gently drop your chin to your chest.
- Slowly roll your head to the right, bringing your right ear toward your right shoulder.
- Continue the circular motion, rolling your head to the back, then to the left, and finally back to the starting position.
- Repeat the motion in the opposite direction.
- Perform 5-10 neck rolls in each direction.

2. Arm Circles:

- Stand with your feet shoulder-width apart.
- Extend your arms out to the sides at shoulder height.

- Begin making small circles with your arms, gradually increasing the size of the circles.
- After 10-15 seconds, reverse the direction of the circles.
- Continue for another 10-15 seconds.

3. Shoulder Rolls:

- Stand with your feet shoulder-width apart.
- Relax your arms at your sides.
- Slowly roll your shoulders forward in a circular motion for 10-15 seconds.
- Reverse the direction and roll your shoulders backward for another 10-15 seconds.

4. Spinal Flexion and Extension:

- Stand with your feet hip-width apart.
- Interlace your fingers and extend your arms in front of you.
- Inhale as you arch your back, lifting your chest and looking up.
- Exhale as you round your spine, tucking your chin toward your chest.

- Repeat this movement, flowing between spinal extension and flexion for 30 seconds.

5. Standing Side Stretch:

- Stand with your feet hip-width apart.
- Reach your right arm overhead and bend your body to the left, creating a side stretch.
- Hold the stretch for 15-20 seconds.
- Return to an upright position.
- Repeat the stretch on the other side.

6. Hip Circles:

- Stand with your feet hip-width apart.
- Place your hands on your hips.
- Begin making small circles with your hips, rotating them clockwise for 10-15 seconds.
- Reverse the direction and rotate your hips counterclockwise for another 10-15 seconds.

7. Leg Swings:

- Stand near a wall or other support for balance.
- Swing your right leg forward and backward in a controlled motion.

-   Perform 10-15 swings with your right leg.

-   Switch to your left leg and repeat.

8. Ankle Circles:

-   Sit on the floor with your legs extended.

-   Lift one foot off the ground and make clockwise and counterclockwise circles with your ankle.

-   Perform 10-15 ankle circles in each direction with each foot.

These warm-up exercises help prepare your body for the specific movements and challenges of Wall Pilates. Perform these stretches and movements mindfully and gradually, paying attention to your body's response.

Once you've completed your warm-up, you'll be ready to transition into your Wall Pilates practice with a reduced risk of injury and improved mobility.

Understanding Your Body's Alignment

Understanding your body's alignment is crucial in Wall Pilates, as proper alignment is at the core of this exercise method.

Maintaining correct alignment ensures that you're engaging the right muscles, prevents strain or injury, and helps you make the most of your Wall Pilates practice. In this section, we'll explore the fundamental principles of body alignment in Wall Pilates:

The Importance of Alignment:

Proper alignment in Wall Pilates is about positioning your body in a way that supports efficient and safe movement. When your body is in the correct alignment, you'll experience the following benefits:

1. Optimal Muscle Engagement: Correct alignment allows you to engage the targeted muscles effectively, leading to better strength development and toning.

2. Reduced Strain: Proper alignment minimizes stress on joints, ligaments, and muscles, reducing the risk of injury.

3. Enhanced Balance and Stability: Maintaining alignment is essential for good balance and stability, which are central to Wall Pilates.

4. Improved Posture: Regular practice of proper alignment in Wall Pilates can lead to better posture in your daily life.

Key Principles of Body Alignment in Wall Pilates:

1. Neutral Spine: In Wall Pilates, neutral spine is a fundamental concept. This means maintaining the natural curve of the spine, which consists of a slight arch in the lower back (lumbar curve), a gentle curve in the upper back (thoracic curve), and a slight forward curve in the neck (cervical curve). Neutral spine is the ideal position for most exercises as it ensures the even distribution of force along the spine.

2. Pelvic Alignment: Your pelvis plays a significant role in alignment. In Wall Pilates, you aim to keep your pelvis level and stable, avoiding excessive tilting or rotation. The alignment of the pelvis influences the position of the spine and, subsequently, the entire body.

3. Ribcage Position: Keep your ribcage relaxed and avoid over-arching or thrusting it forward. The ribcage should be positioned so that it's gently pulled down toward the pelvis, maintaining a connection between the lower and upper abdominals.

4. Shoulder Placement: Ensure that your shoulders are relaxed and away from your ears.

They should be in a neutral position, not hunched forward or pulled back excessively.

Proper shoulder placement is essential for maintaining a stable spine and preventing tension in the neck and upper back.

5. Head and Neck Alignment: Keep your head aligned with your spine. Avoid jutting your chin forward or dropping it excessively. Maintain a neutral head position with your gaze forward, and avoid straining the neck.

Wall as Your Reference Point:

The wall is a valuable reference point for alignment in Wall Pilates. As you perform exercises, use the wall to guide your positioning. For example:

- In exercises where your back is against the wall, make sure your spine is in contact with the wall from the tailbone to the head.
- For standing exercises, use the wall to maintain proper posture and ensure that your weight is evenly distributed between your feet.

Breathing and Alignment:

Breathing is an integral part of Pilates and plays a role in alignment. In Wall Pilates, coordinated breathing helps support the alignment of your spine.

Typically, you'll inhale to prepare for a movement and exhale to execute it. Breath control promotes core engagement and assists in maintaining alignment throughout exercises.

Understanding and practicing proper body alignment is an ongoing process. It's helpful to start with the basics and gradually incorporate alignment principles into more complex exercises.

Over time, focusing on alignment will become second nature, enhancing the safety and effectiveness of your Wall Pilates practice.

If you're new to Wall Pilates, consider working with a certified instructor who can provide guidance and corrections to ensure your alignment is accurate.

CHAPTER THREE

Fundamental Wall Pilates Exercises

Wall Pilates, an innovative approach to the classical Pilates method, marries the principles of mind-body connection, core engagement, and proper alignment with the unique support and resistance of a wall.

In this section, we will delve into the world of Wall Pilates and explore the fundamental exercises that form the backbone of this dynamic and holistic fitness practice.

The Essence of Wall Pilates

Pilates, developed by Joseph Pilates in the early 20th century, is renowned for its focus on mindful movement, core strength, and balanced development of the body.

Wall Pilates preserves these core principles while introducing the wall as a steadfast partner in your fitness journey.

The wall provides support, stability, and the opportunity to deepen your practice by incorporating resistance, challenging your balance, and enhancing your flexibility.

Pilates Basics

Before we dive into the specifics of Wall Pilates exercises, let's revisit the foundational principles that underpin both classical and Wall Pilates:

- Concentration: Pilates is not about mindless repetitions but rather a mindful engagement with each movement. Concentration is key to performing exercises with precision and control.
- Control: Controlled movements are a hallmark of Pilates. By moving deliberately, you avoid unnecessary tension and ensure proper muscle engagement.
- Centering: At the core of Pilates is the centering concept, emphasizing the engagement of the core muscles, including the abdominals and lower back, to provide stability and strength.
- Precision: Each exercise should be executed with precision and alignment. Proper form is critical to maximize the benefits and minimize the risk of injury.

- Breath: Coordinating your breath with movement is integral to Pilates. Inhaling to prepare and exhaling during the exertion helps enhance your control, concentration, and stamina.
- Flow: Flowing movements contribute to a sense of harmony and continuity in your practice, making transitions between exercises graceful and seamless.

Wall Pilates embodies these principles while incorporating the wall as a supportive and guiding element, allowing you to deepen your mind-body connection and improve your overall fitness.

The Benefits of Wall Pilates

Wall Pilates offers a wealth of advantages, making it a sought-after exercise method for individuals of various fitness levels and backgrounds. Here are some of the key benefits you can expect from practicing Wall Pilates:

1. Enhanced Core Strength: The wall provides resistance and support for core-focused exercises, helping you build a strong and stable core, which is essential for overall body strength and posture.

2. Improved Posture: Wall Pilates emphasizes proper alignment, helping you develop better posture and alignment awareness that can carry over into your daily life.

3. Increased Flexibility: Through controlled and deliberate movements, Wall Pilates contributes to improved flexibility and range of motion, reducing muscle tightness and stiffness.

4. Balanced Muscle Development: Wall Pilates exercises are designed to work multiple muscle groups simultaneously, promoting balanced muscle development and a more toned physique.

5. Better Balance and Stability: The wall provides a stable platform for exercises that challenge your balance and coordination, enhancing your functional fitness.

6. Low-Impact Nature: Wall Pilates is gentle on the joints, making it accessible to individuals of various ages and fitness levels.

7. Mind-Body Connection: Like traditional Pilates, Wall Pilates fosters a strong mind-body connection, promoting mindfulness, concentration, and self-awareness.

8. Resistance Training: The wall can serve as a source of resistance, allowing you to progressively increase the intensity of your exercises to build strength and endurance.

In essence, Wall Pilates provides a comprehensive and balanced approach to fitness that targets your body, mind, and overall well-being.

Your Journey Begins

As we embark on this exploration of Wall Pilates exercises, you'll discover how the wall can become your steadfast partner in your pursuit of strength, balance, and flexibility. It's a unique and empowering approach to holistic fitness that will guide you towards a deeper connection with your body and a heightened sense of well-being.

Whether you're a seasoned Pilates practitioner seeking a fresh perspective or a newcomer eager to unlock the potential of Wall Pilates, this journey is sure to enrich your understanding of your body's capabilities and the profound impact of mindful movement. The wall is your ally in this quest, offering support, resistance, and a source of inspiration for your physical and mental growth.

Let's step up to the wall and embrace the transformative power of Wall Pilates.

Wall Squats and Leg Toning

Wall squats are an excellent Wall Pilates exercise that can help you tone and strengthen your legs while improving your balance and stability. This exercise combines the benefits of traditional squats with the unique support of the wall, creating a challenging yet rewarding workout for your lower body.

Wall Squats: Step-by-Step

Follow these step-by-step instructions to perform Wall Squats effectively:

1. Set Up: Stand with your back against a smooth, clean wall. Ensure that your feet are hip-width apart and your toes are pointing forward.

2. Align Your Spine: Focus on maintaining a neutral spine. Keep your shoulders relaxed and your head in line with your spine.

3. Lower Your Body: Inhale and start to bend your knees, slowly lowering your body toward the wall. Keep your back in contact with the wall throughout the movement.

4. Thighs Parallel:

Continue to lower your body until your thighs are parallel to the ground. Your knees should be directly above your ankles.

5. Hold and Breathe: Hold this position for a moment, focusing on your breath. Exhale as you hold the squat.

6. Push and Stand: Exhale and push through your heels to return to the starting position, fully extending your legs.

7. Repeat: Perform 10-15 repetitions of Wall Squats. As you become more comfortable with the exercise, you can increase the number of repetitions or add resistance for added intensity.

Tips for Effective Wall Squats:

- Ensure that your knees are aligned with your ankles and that they do not extend past your toes during the squat to protect your knees.

- Keep your weight centered over your heels to maintain proper balance and reduce stress on your knees.
- Engage your core muscles to support your lower back and maintain a stable spine.
- Focus on the quality of each repetition rather than the quantity. Performing Wall Squats with proper form is more important than the number of repetitions.

Leg Toning with Wall Squats:

Wall squats are an effective exercise for toning and strengthening your legs, targeting several major muscle groups, including:

1. Quadriceps: Wall squats heavily engage your quadriceps, the muscles on the front of your thighs. As you lower your body, these muscles work to extend your knees and lift your body back up.

2. Hamstrings: Your hamstrings, located on the back of your thighs, play a role in controlling your descent and assisting in the return to the starting position.

3. Glutes: Wall squats activate your gluteal muscles, or the muscles in your buttocks, to help you maintain an upright posture and support your pelvis.

4. Calves: As you push through your heels to stand up, your calf muscles are engaged, contributing to the overall strength and tone of your lower legs.

5. Adductors and Abductors: The inner and outer thigh muscles (adductors and abductors) help stabilize your knees and hips during the exercise, enhancing leg toning and balance.

Incorporating Wall Squats into your Wall Pilates routine can lead to improved leg strength, enhanced muscle tone, and greater overall lower body fitness. Additionally, these exercises are gentle on the joints and can be adjusted to suit various fitness levels, making them a versatile choice for anyone looking to tone and strengthen their legs.

Wall Angels for Posture and Flexibility

Wall Angels, also known as Wall Angels or Snow Angels, are an effective exercise for improving posture, increasing flexibility, and enhancing upper body mobility.

This Wall Pilates exercise is designed to open up the chest, strengthen the upper back and shoulder muscles, and promote better alignment. Wall Angels can be particularly beneficial for individuals who spend long hours sitting at a desk or have postural issues.

Wall Angels: Step-by-Step

Follow these step-by-step instructions to perform Wall Angels effectively:

1. Set Up: Stand with your back against a smooth, clean wall. Your heels, buttocks, upper back, and head should all be in contact with the wall. Position your feet hip-width apart and keep your knees slightly bent to avoid locking them.

2. Arm Position: Start with your arms bent at a 90-degree angle, with your elbows at shoulder height and your palms facing forward. Keep your arms pressed against the wall throughout the exercise.

3. Begin the Movement: Slowly slide your arms upward along the wall, keeping your elbows and wrists in contact with the wall. Continue to raise your arms as high as your shoulder flexibility allows,

aiming to bring your arms overhead without letting them leave the wall.

4. Full Extension: At the highest point, your arms should be fully extended overhead, forming a "Y" shape with your body.

5. Reverse the Movement: Reverse the motion by sliding your arms back down to the starting position. Keep your elbows, wrists, and palms in contact with the wall as you lower your arms.

6. Repeat: Perform 10-15 repetitions of Wall Angels. Focus on smooth and controlled movements, paying attention to your breath.

Tips for Effective Wall Angels:

- Maintain proper alignment with your entire back, including your head, in contact with the wall. If you have difficulty keeping your head against the wall, use a small cushion or towel roll for support.

- Focus on the quality of the movement, ensuring that your arms remain in contact with the wall throughout. It's more important to perform the exercise correctly than to achieve a high range of motion.

- Engage your core muscles to support your lower back and pelvis throughout the exercise.

- Breathe naturally and consistently as you perform Wall Angels. Inhale as you raise your arms, and exhale as you lower them.

Benefits of Wall Angels:

Wall Angels offer numerous benefits for your posture, flexibility, and upper body:

1. Improved Posture: Wall Angels help align your spine, open up your chest, and strengthen the upper back muscles, promoting better posture and reducing the risk of rounded shoulders and forward head posture.

2. Increased Flexibility: The controlled movement of Wall Angels enhances the flexibility of your shoulder joints and the surrounding muscles, allowing for greater range of motion in your arms.

3. Upper Body Strength: This exercise engages the muscles of the upper back, shoulders, and arms, contributing to upper body strength and toning.

4. Enhanced Mobility: Wall Angels improve the mobility of your shoulder girdle, making everyday activities, such as reaching overhead, more comfortable and fluid.

5. Stress Relief: The rhythmic and controlled motion of Wall Angels can have a calming and stress-relieving effect, making them a great addition to your relaxation routine.

Incorporating Wall Angels into your Wall Pilates practice can have a transformative impact on your posture, flexibility, and upper body strength.

Regularly performing this exercise can help counteract the negative effects of prolonged sitting and improve your overall upper body mobility and alignment.

Wall Roll Downs for Core Strength

Wall Roll Downs are a powerful Wall Pilates exercise that targets core strength while also improving flexibility, posture, and spinal mobility. This exercise is designed to engage the abdominal muscles, particularly the lower abdominals, as well as the muscles along the spine, helping you build a strong and stable core while promoting a healthy spine.

Here's a step-by-step guide on how to perform Wall Roll Downs effectively:

1. Set Up:

- Stand with your back against a clean, smooth wall. Ensure that your heels, buttocks, upper back, and head are all in contact with the wall.
- Your feet should be hip-width apart and your knees slightly bent to avoid locking them.
- **3. Arm Position:** Place your arms by your sides with your palms facing forward and your shoulders relaxed.

3. Inhale and Prepare: Inhale deeply to prepare for the movement. Allow your ribcage to expand as you breathe in.

4. Begin the Roll Down:

- Exhale and start to roll down your spine, articulating each vertebra as you go.
- Keep your head in line with your spine, and let your chin move toward your chest.
- Continue to round your spine as you move down, aiming to bring your hands as close to the ground as your flexibility allows.

5. Hold the Position: Once you've reached your maximum stretch or a comfortable point, hold the position for a few breaths. Ensure that your back, head, and arms remain in contact with the wall.

6. Begin the Roll Up: Inhale and start to roll back up, reversing the movement. Articulate each vertebra as you return to the starting position.

7. Finish the Roll Up: Continue the movement until you're fully upright with your head, upper back, and buttocks in contact with the wall.

8. Repeat: Perform 8-10 repetitions of Wall Roll Downs. Focus on controlled and deliberate movements, and coordinate your breath with each phase of the exercise.

Tips for Effective Wall Roll Downs:

- Maintain consistent contact between your back, head, and arms with the wall throughout the entire movement. If your flexibility is limited, go only as far as comfortable.

- Engage your core muscles, particularly the lower abdominals, to support your spine as you roll down and back up.

- Keep your shoulders relaxed and your neck in a neutral position to avoid strain.

- Breathe rhythmically, inhaling to prepare and exhaling as you roll down and inhaling as you roll back up.

Benefits of Wall Roll Downs:

Wall Roll Downs offer numerous benefits for core strength and overall well-being:

1. Core Strength: This exercise is highly effective at engaging and strengthening the core muscles, especially the lower abdominals.

2. Spinal Mobility: Wall Roll Downs promote mobility and flexibility in the spine, reducing the risk of stiffness and enhancing posture.

3. Posture Improvement: By reinforcing spinal alignment, Wall Roll Downs contribute to better posture and body awareness.

4. Breath Control: The coordinated breath in this exercise helps improve breath control, allowing for better oxygen exchange during exercise.

5. Relaxation and Stress Reduction: The rhythmic and controlled nature of Wall Roll Downs can have a calming effect, making them a valuable addition to stress-relief routines.

Incorporating Wall Roll Downs into your Wall Pilates practice can help you build a strong core, maintain a flexible spine, and foster better posture. Whether you're seeking core strength, flexibility, or an improved sense of well-being, Wall Roll Downs offer a comprehensive solution that can be tailored to your fitness level and goals.

Wall Leg Circles and Hip Mobility

Wall Leg Circles are a beneficial Wall Pilates exercise that focuses on improving hip mobility while also engaging the core muscles. This exercise can help enhance flexibility, strengthen the hip muscles, and promote overall lower body mobility. Here's a step-by-step guide on how to perform Wall Leg Circles effectively:

1. Set Up:

- Stand with your back against a clean, smooth wall. Ensure that your heels, buttocks, upper back, and head are all in contact with the wall.

- Your feet should be hip-width apart, and your knees should be slightly bent to prevent them from locking.

2. Arm Position: Place your arms by your sides with your palms facing forward. This provides balance and stability during the exercise.

3. Inhale and Prepare: Inhale deeply to prepare for the movement, allowing your ribcage to expand as you breathe in.

4. Start the Leg Circle: Exhale and raise one leg in front of you, keeping it straight and parallel to the ground. Engage your core muscles to support your lower back.

5. Circle Your Leg: Begin to circle your raised leg in a clockwise direction. Your circle should be controlled and deliberate. Keep your leg close to the wall without touching it.

6. Reverse Direction: After completing several clockwise circles, reverse the direction of the leg circle and continue circling in a counterclockwise direction.

7. Complete the Leg Circle: After performing both clockwise and counterclockwise leg circles, lower your leg to the starting position with control.

8. Switch Legs: Perform the same sequence of leg circles with your opposite leg.

9. Repeat: Continue the exercise by alternating legs. Aim to perform 8-10 circles in each direction with each leg.

Tips for Effective Wall Leg Circles:

- Keep your core engaged and your lower back in contact with the wall to support your spine and maintain stability.
- Maintain a slow and controlled pace while performing leg circles. The focus should be on form and precision rather than speed.
- Breathe rhythmically throughout the exercise, inhaling as you prepare to lift your leg and exhaling as you circle it.

Benefits of Wall Leg Circles:

Wall Leg Circles offer a range of advantages for hip mobility, core engagement, and overall well-being:

1. Improved Hip Mobility: These circles help enhance the range of motion in your hip joints, making daily movements easier and reducing the risk of hip stiffness.

2. Core Engagement: Wall Leg Circles require core stability and strength to control the movement of the leg, contributing to better core engagement.

3. Flexibility: This exercise promotes flexibility in the hips and hamstrings, reducing the risk of muscle tightness.

4. Balance and Coordination: Performing leg circles in a controlled manner can improve your balance and coordination, enhancing overall mobility.

5. Stress Reduction: The focused and deliberate nature of Wall Leg Circles can have a calming effect, making them a valuable addition to stress-relief routines.

Incorporating Wall Leg Circles into your Wall Pilates practice can help you improve hip mobility, strengthen the core, and experience greater overall lower body flexibility.

Whether you're looking to enhance your hip range of motion, achieve better core engagement, or simply increase your lower body flexibility, Wall Leg Circles provide a versatile exercise to help you achieve your goals.

Wall Bridging for Glute and Hamstring Activation

Wall Bridging is a highly effective Wall Pilates exercise that targets the gluteal muscles and hamstrings while engaging the core. This exercise helps to build strength in the lower body, particularly the glutes, and enhances hamstring flexibility. Wall Bridging also supports spinal mobility and stability. Here's a step-by-step guide on how to perform Wall Bridging effectively:

1. Set Up:

- Lie on your back with your feet flat on the floor and your knees bent. Your feet should be hip-width apart and close to the wall.
- Ensure that your arms are by your sides with your palms facing down, and your head is resting comfortably on the floor.

2. Engage Your Core: Before starting the movement, engage your core muscles by drawing your navel toward your spine. This core engagement will support your lower back throughout the exercise.

3. Start the Bridging:

- Exhale as you press your feet into the floor, lifting your hips off the ground.
- Continue to lift your hips until your body forms a straight line from your shoulders to your knees. Your feet and shoulders should remain on the floor, while your weight is supported by your feet and upper back.

4. Hold the Bridge: At the top of the bridge, pause for a moment and engage your glutes and hamstrings to maintain stability.

5. Lower Your Hips: Inhale and slowly lower your hips back to the floor, one vertebra at a time. Begin with your upper back, then your middle back, and finally your lower back.

6. Repeat: Perform 10-12 repetitions of Wall Bridging. Focus on controlled and deliberate movements while coordinating your breath with each phase of the exercise.

Tips for Effective Wall Bridging:

- Keep your feet and knees hip-width apart throughout the exercise to maintain proper alignment.
- Focus on maintaining a straight line from your shoulders to your knees when you're at the top of the bridge.
- Breathe rhythmically, exhaling as you lift your hips and inhaling as you lower them.

Benefits of Wall Bridging:

Wall Bridging offers a range of advantages for glute and hamstring activation, core engagement, and overall well-being:

1. Glute Activation: This exercise effectively targets the gluteal muscles, helping to build strength and tone in the buttocks.

2. Hamstring Engagement: Wall Bridging also engages the hamstrings, contributing to improved flexibility and strength in the back of the thighs.

3. Core Strength: To maintain the bridge position, the core muscles must work to stabilize the spine, enhancing core strength and stability.

4. Spinal Mobility: Wall Bridging supports spinal mobility, especially in the lower back, which can be beneficial for individuals with sedentary jobs or activities.

5. Posture Improvement: By strengthening the core and the muscles that support the spine, Wall Bridging can help improve overall posture.

Incorporating Wall Bridging into your Wall Pilates practice can help you activate and strengthen your glutes and hamstrings, engage your core, and promote spinal mobility.

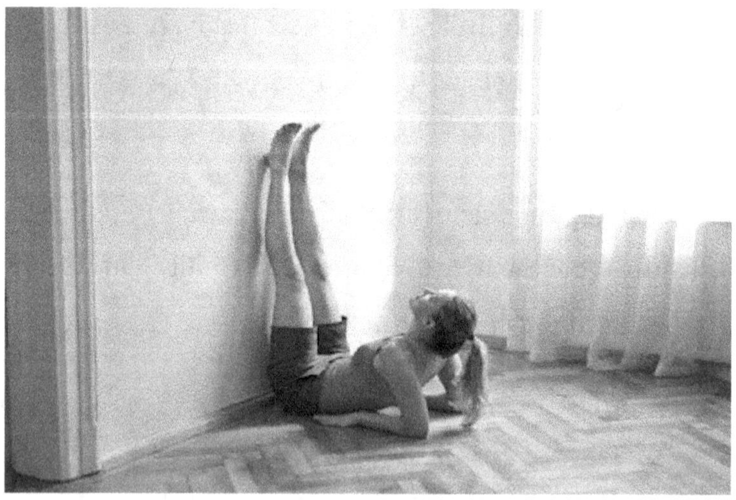

CHAPTER FOUR

Progressing in Wall Pilates

Wall Pilates, a unique and innovative fusion of classical Pilates principles and the support of a wall, offers a transformative path to strength, balance, and overall well-being. In this comprehensive guide, we will explore the art of progressing in Wall Pilates, enabling you to take your practice to new heights and experience the full spectrum of its benefits.

The Foundations of Wall Pilates

Before delving into the realms of progression, let's revisit the core principles that make Wall Pilates a captivating and effective fitness methodology:

- Mind-Body Connection: Wall Pilates places a strong emphasis on the connection between your mind and body. It encourages you to be present in every movement, fostering mindfulness and a deeper understanding of your body.

- Core Engagement: Central to Wall Pilates is the activation of the core muscles, particularly the abdominal and lower back muscles.

A strong core provides the foundation for stability, strength, and graceful movement.

- Alignment: Proper alignment is crucial in Wall Pilates. It helps prevent strain, optimize muscle engagement, and contribute to improved posture. The wall serves as a reference point for alignment, ensuring that your body remains in the correct position.

- Breath Control: Coordinating your breath with movement is an essential component of Wall Pilates. Proper breathing patterns enhance control, focus, and the efficiency of your exercises.

- Controlled Movements: Wall Pilates emphasizes the quality of movement over quantity. Controlled, precise movements are paramount to gain the full benefits of each exercise.

- Flow: Fluidity and flow between movements are core principles of Wall Pilates. Smooth transitions enhance the harmony of your practice.

The Journey of Progression

Progression in Wall Pilates is about evolving and challenging your practice as you grow stronger and more experienced. It allows you to push your boundaries, deepen your connection with your body, and uncover new dimensions of fitness. As you progress, you'll encounter three key elements that define your journey:

1. Increasing Complexity

At the heart of progression in Wall Pilates is the gradual introduction of more complex exercises. As you become proficient in foundational movements, you can explore variations and advanced techniques that target different muscle groups and enhance your skills. The beauty of Wall Pilates lies in its versatility, offering a vast repertoire of exercises that can be adapted to your level of proficiency.

For example, you may begin with basic Wall Squats and progress to Single-Leg Wall Squats, which challenge your balance and strength more intensively. Similarly, Wall Angels can evolve into Wall Angel Circles, which involve dynamic movements and a higher degree of coordination.

2. Increased Intensity

Progression also involves increasing the intensity of your exercises. You can achieve this through various means, such as adjusting the number of repetitions, incorporating resistance bands or weights, or extending the duration of holds. By intensifying your workouts, you'll stimulate muscle growth, endurance, and functional fitness.

For instance, Wall Roll Downs can be made more challenging by extending the time spent in the rolled-down position or by adding resistance bands to increase the workload on your core and spine. This enhanced intensity not only builds strength but also deepens your mind-body connection.

3. Refinement and Precision

As you progress, you'll refine your movements and enhance your precision. This refinement is about perfecting your alignment, breathing, and execution of exercises. It's the art of making each movement more efficient, ensuring that your body is working optimally, and preventing imbalances or strain.

For instance, Wall Bridging can be refined by paying careful attention to the articulation of each vertebra when lifting and lowering the hips. By honing this skill, you can optimize the benefits of the exercise and maintain proper spinal alignment.

The Benefits of Progression

Progressing in Wall Pilates offers a host of benefits that extend beyond physical fitness. These advantages include:

- Enhanced Strength: Progression helps you build greater strength, targeting specific muscle groups and improving overall functional fitness.

- Deeper Mind-Body Connection: As you refine your practice and increase complexity, you'll develop a profound connection with your body, fostering mindfulness and self-awareness.

- Postural Improvement: Progression enhances your alignment and posture, reducing the risk of postural issues caused by modern sedentary lifestyles.

- Better Mobility and Flexibility: As exercises become more challenging, your flexibility and mobility are tested and improved, contributing to enhanced range of motion.

- Increased Confidence: Achieving new milestones in your practice boosts your self-confidence and self-efficacy.

- Stress Reduction: The focused and mindful nature of Wall Pilates progression can provide a sense of calm and stress relief.

Your Journey Awaits

The journey of progression in Wall Pilates is an empowering and fulfilling endeavor. Whether you're a seasoned practitioner seeking new challenges or a newcomer eager to explore the world of Wall Pilates, the path of progression is a gateway to holistic well-being.

By increasing complexity, intensity, and precision in your practice, you'll unlock the full potential of Wall Pilates, shaping not only your body but also your mind and spirit. So, step up to the wall and embark on a journey of self-discovery and transformation through Wall Pilates progression.

Advanced Wall Pilates Techniques

Advanced Wall Pilates Techniques are the next level of Wall Pilates practice, designed for individuals who have a solid foundation in the basic and intermediate exercises and are ready to further challenge themselves. These advanced techniques take your strength, flexibility, and mind-body connection to new heights, offering a holistic and rewarding fitness experience.

1. Wall Piston Splits

Execution: Start in a seated position on the floor with your back against the wall and your legs straight. Lift one leg off the ground, keeping it as straight as possible. Slowly slide the lifted leg up and down the wall, aiming to maintain a straight leg throughout. This exercise challenges hamstring flexibility and strengthens the core.

Key Benefits: Wall Piston Splits enhance flexibility and strengthen the hamstrings and core. The support of the wall provides stability for safe execution.

2. Wall Plank Variations

Execution: Begin in a plank position facing away from the wall, with your hands on the floor and your feet against the wall. You can perform various plank variations, such as shoulder taps, leg lifts, or knee tucks, to intensify the core and upper body engagement. Wall Plank Variations enhance strength and stability, especially in the shoulders and core.

Key Benefits: These advanced plank variations challenge your balance and upper body strength while still providing a supportive wall base.

3. Wall Teaser

Execution: Sit on the floor with your back to the wall and your knees bent. Place your feet flat on the floor and your hands on the ground for support. Lift your feet off the ground, extending your legs and balancing on your tailbone. Roll backward, extending your legs up the wall, and then roll back up to a balanced position. Wall Teasers require a strong core and balance.

Key Benefits: Wall Teasers improve core strength and balance, targeting both the abdominal and hip flexor muscles. The wall provides support and guidance for the exercise.

4. Wall Scissor Variations

Execution: Lie on your back with your buttocks close to the wall and your legs extended. Lift one leg up and rest it against the wall while the other leg hovers just above the ground. Perform scissor-like movements, switching the position of your legs in a controlled manner.

Wall Scissor Variations challenge core stability, lower abdominal strength, and hip flexibility.

Key Benefits: These advanced variations of the scissor exercise intensify core engagement and promote greater lower body flexibility.

5. Wall Handstand Progression

Execution: Begin in a plank position facing the wall, with your hands close to the wall and your feet resting on it. Walk your feet up the wall until your body is in an inverted V position. To progress further, practice lifting one leg off the wall or attempting freestanding handstands with the wall as support.

Key Benefits: Wall Handstand Progression enhances upper body strength, balance, and coordination. It is a valuable step toward achieving a full handstand.

6. Wall Roll Ups

Execution: Sit with your back against the wall, your legs extended, and your feet flexed. Begin to roll backward, one vertebra at a time, and then roll back up to a seated position with control. Wall Roll Ups challenge core strength, spinal mobility, and body control.

Key Benefits: Wall Roll Ups are a more advanced variation of the classic Pilates exercise, promoting core strength and spine articulation while providing support from the wall.

7. Wall Leg Circles with Resistance

Execution: Perform Wall Leg Circles, but this time add resistance by using an elastic band around your ankles. The resistance intensifies the challenge to your hip muscles, hamstrings, and core.

Key Benefits: Adding resistance to Wall Leg Circles increases the difficulty and enhances lower body strength and flexibility.

These advanced Wall Pilates techniques require a strong foundation in the basic and intermediate exercises, as well as a deep understanding of proper alignment, breath control, and core engagement.

It's essential to approach advanced techniques with caution and gradually progress as your strength and skills improve.

If you're new to advanced Wall Pilates exercises, consider working with a certified instructor who can provide guidance and ensure your safety while advancing your practice.

Combining Exercises for Full-Body Workouts

Combining Wall Pilates exercises for full-body workouts can be an effective way to target multiple muscle groups, enhance overall strength, and promote flexibility and balance.

Here are some sample full-body workout routines that incorporate a variety of Wall Pilates exercises. Remember to warm up before starting any workout and consult with a fitness professional if you're new to these exercises.

Full-Body Workout Routine 1: Intermediate Level

This workout combines both upper and lower body exercises and is suitable for individuals with an intermediate level of Wall Pilates experience.

1. Wall Squats - 3 sets of 12 reps: Focus on proper form and control while performing Wall Squats. Engage your core and keep your back against the wall for support.

2. Wall Angels - 3 sets of 10 reps: Wall Angels help improve posture and enhance upper body mobility. Perform smooth and controlled movements.

3. Wall Leg Circles - 3 sets of 10 reps per leg: Wall Leg Circles target the lower body and improve hip mobility. Ensure that your core is engaged for stability.

4. Wall Roll Downs - 3 sets of 8 reps: Wall Roll Downs engage your core and spinal mobility. Pay attention to the articulation of your spine during the exercise.

5. Wall Bridging - 3 sets of 10 reps: Wall Bridging focuses on the glutes and hamstrings. Lift your hips off the ground to create a straight line from your shoulders to your knees.

6. Wall Angels - 3 sets of 10 reps (cooldown): Finish with another set of Wall Angels to promote post-workout relaxation and improved upper body mobility.

Full-Body Workout Routine 2: Advanced Level

For those with a more advanced level of Wall Pilates experience, this workout incorporates challenging exercises that target both the upper and lower body.

1. Wall Piston Splits - 3 sets of 8 reps per leg: Wall Piston Splits challenge hamstring flexibility and core strength. Keep your back against the wall as you perform the exercise.

2. Wall Plank Variations - 3 sets of 30 seconds each: Incorporate various Wall Plank Variations, such as shoulder taps, leg lifts, or knee tucks, to intensify core and upper body engagement.

3. Wall Teasers - 3 sets of 8 reps: Wall Teasers focus on the core and balance. Roll back and forth while maintaining a V-sit position.

4. Wall Scissor Variations - 3 sets of 10 reps per leg: Wall Scissor Variations challenge core stability and lower body flexibility. Perform scissor-like movements with precision.

5. Wall Handstand Progression - 3 sets of 30 seconds (if applicable): For advanced individuals, attempt Wall Handstand Progression to target the upper body, balance, and coordination.

6. Wall Roll Ups - 3 sets of 8 reps: Wall Roll Ups are an advanced variation of the classic exercise, engaging the core and promoting spinal mobility.

7. Wall Leg Circles with Resistance - 3 sets of 10 reps per leg: Use an elastic band for resistance during Wall Leg Circles to intensify the challenge to your lower body.

Remember to maintain proper alignment, engage your core, and breathe consistently throughout these exercises. It's crucial to perform each movement with control and precision to maximize the benefits and reduce the risk of injury.

Adjust the number of sets and repetitions based on your fitness level, and gradually progress as you become more comfortable with these advanced exercises. Always prioritize safety and listen to your body during your Wall Pilates workouts.

Creating Your Own Wall Pilates Routine

Creating your own Wall Pilates routine allows you to tailor your workout to your specific goals, fitness level, and preferences.

Whether you're looking to build strength, improve flexibility, enhance posture, or simply enjoy a well-rounded fitness routine, here's a step-by-step guide to help you design a personalized Wall Pilates routine:

1. Determine Your Goals:

Begin by identifying your fitness objectives. Are you aiming to strengthen your core, improve flexibility, or work on your posture? Knowing your goals will guide the selection of exercises for your routine.

2. Assess Your Fitness Level:

Consider your current fitness level. If you're new to Wall Pilates, it's advisable to start with basic exercises and gradually progress to more advanced ones as you build strength and confidence.

3. Warm-Up:

A proper warm-up is essential to prepare your body for exercise. Incorporate dynamic movements like leg swings, arm circles, and gentle stretches to increase blood flow and flexibility.

4. Exercise Selection:

Choose a variety of Wall Pilates exercises that align with your goals and fitness level. Aim to include exercises that target different muscle groups and movement patterns for a balanced workout. For example:

- Core Strength: Include exercises like Wall Squats, Wall Roll Downs, and Wall Teasers.
- Flexibility: Incorporate Wall Leg Circles and Wall Handstand Progression.
- Posture Improvement: Add Wall Angels and Wall Bridging to your routine.

5. Create a Sequence:

Arrange your chosen exercises in a logical sequence. Begin with exercises that engage your core and gradually move on to exercises that focus on other muscle groups. This helps prevent fatigue and ensures a well-rounded workout.

6. Sets and Repetitions:

Determine the number of sets and repetitions for each exercise. For beginners, start with 2-3 sets of 8-12 repetitions for each exercise. As you progress, you can increase the number of sets and repetitions.

7. Rest Intervals:

Incorporate short rest intervals between sets and exercises to allow for recovery. Aim for 30-60 seconds of rest between sets and 1-2 minutes between different exercises.

8. Cool-Down:

After completing your exercises, perform a cool-down routine that includes static stretching. Stretch the major muscle groups you worked during your routine, holding each stretch for 15-30 seconds.

9. Breathing:

Pay attention to your breath throughout the routine. Inhale as you prepare for a movement and exhale as you execute it. Proper breathing enhances control and engagement of your core muscles.

10. Progression:

As you become more comfortable with your routine, consider adding more advanced exercises or increasing the intensity by adding resistance, like resistance bands or weights.

11. Consistency:

Consistency is key to seeing progress. Aim to practice your Wall Pilates routine at least 2-3 times per week to experience the benefits and improvements.

12. Listen to Your Body:

Always listen to your body and modify or skip exercises if you experience discomfort or pain. Safety should be your top priority.

13. Seek Guidance:

If you're new to Wall Pilates, consider taking classes with a certified instructor or working with a fitness professional to ensure you're performing exercises correctly and safely.

Remember that creating your own Wall Pilates routine is a flexible and adaptable process. It should evolve as your fitness level and goals change.

By following these steps and customizing your routine to suit your unique needs, you can enjoy the full benefits of Wall Pilates while tailoring your practice to meet your individual fitness aspirations.

Tracking Your Progress and Setting Goals

Tracking your progress and setting goals in Wall Pilates is a vital part of maintaining motivation, measuring your achievements, and continually improving your practice.

Here's how to effectively track your progress and establish achievable goals in Wall Pilates:

1. Establish Clear Goals:

Start by defining your goals. Be specific about what you want to achieve with your Wall Pilates practice. Examples of goals might include improving core strength, increasing flexibility, correcting posture, or mastering a specific advanced exercise. Setting clear, measurable objectives is the foundation for progress tracking.

2. Assess Your Baseline:

Before embarking on your Wall Pilates journey, assess your current fitness level. Note your strengths and weaknesses, flexibility, and any postural issues. This baseline assessment provides a starting point for measuring your progress.

3. Create a Progress Journal:

Maintain a dedicated journal or digital record of your Wall Pilates practice. Include details such as the exercises you perform, sets and repetitions, any modifications or variations, and how you felt during and after each session.

4. Track Your Strength and Flexibility:

Regularly measure and track your strength and flexibility using specific exercises or flexibility tests. For example, you can measure how long you can hold a Wall Plank or track your progress in Wall Leg Circles by monitoring the range of motion of your legs.

5. Set SMART Goals:

Use the SMART goal-setting framework to ensure your goals are Specific, Measurable, Achievable, Relevant, and Time-bound. For instance, rather than saying, "I want to improve my core strength," set a goal like, "I aim to perform 3 sets of 12 Wall Roll Ups with proper form within 3 months."

6. Monitor Your Progress Regularly:

Consistently assess your progress, ideally every few weeks. Revisit your baseline assessments and compare your current abilities to your initial measurements. Evaluate which exercises have become easier and where you've seen improvement.

7. Adjust Your Routine:

Based on your progress, make adjustments to your Wall Pilates routine. If an exercise has become too easy, try a more challenging variation. Conversely, if you're struggling with certain exercises, consider modifying them or seeking guidance from an instructor.

8. Celebrate Milestones:

Recognize and celebrate your achievements along the way. Whether it's mastering a new exercise, holding a position for a longer duration, or noticing improved posture, acknowledging your successes keeps you motivated.

9. Seek Professional Guidance:

Consider working with a certified Wall Pilates instructor who can assess your progress objectively, provide feedback, and offer expert guidance on setting and achieving your goals. They can also assist in designing a tailored routine.

10. Be Patient and Persistent:

Progress in Wall Pilates, as in any fitness discipline, takes time. Understand that results may not be immediately visible, but consistency and perseverance are key. Stay patient and trust the process.

11. Reevaluate and Adjust Goals:

Periodically review your goals to ensure they remain relevant and challenging. As you achieve your initial objectives, set new goals to continue pushing your boundaries and advancing your practice.

12. Listen to Your Body:

While striving to achieve your goals, always prioritize safety and listen to your body. If you experience pain or discomfort, don't hesitate to adjust your routine or seek guidance from a professional.

Tracking your progress and setting goals in Wall Pilates can transform your practice into a dynamic and fulfilling journey of self-improvement. By monitoring your achievements and continuously striving for new milestones, you'll experience the benefits of improved strength, flexibility, posture, and overall well-being.

Maintaining a Consistent Wall Pilates Practice

Maintaining a consistent Wall Pilates practice is essential for reaping the full benefits of this fitness discipline.

Here are some tips to help you stay dedicated and make Wall Pilates a regular part of your routine:

1. Set Clear Goals:

Establish specific, achievable goals that motivate you to continue your Wall Pilates practice. Having a clear sense of purpose can help you stay committed.

2. Create a Schedule:

Plan your Wall Pilates sessions in advance and allocate specific time slots in your weekly schedule. Treating your practice like an appointment can make it easier to prioritize.

3. Choose a Dedicated Space:

Designate a space in your home or gym specifically for Wall Pilates. Having a dedicated area can help you focus and get into the right mindset for your practice.

4. Consistency Over Intensity:

Consistency is more important than intensity. It's better to do shorter sessions regularly than to have sporadic, intense workouts. Even 10-20 minutes of daily practice can yield benefits.

5. Find a Routine That Suits You:

Select a Wall Pilates routine that matches your fitness level and preferences. A routine you enjoy is more likely to become a consistent habit.

6. Mix It Up:

While having a routine is important, don't be afraid to mix up your exercises to prevent boredom and maintain enthusiasm. You can introduce new exercises or variations periodically.

7. Start Slowly:

If you're new to Wall Pilates, begin with a manageable schedule, such as 2-3 sessions per week. Gradually increase the frequency as your body adapts and your motivation grows.

8. Set Reminders:

Use reminders on your phone or a calendar to prompt you to practice. Having a visual or auditory cue can help you remember your scheduled sessions.

9. Include a Friend:

Practicing Wall Pilates with a friend or family member can be motivating and enjoyable. You can keep each other accountable and make it a social activity.

10. Join a Class:

Enroll in a Wall Pilates class or hire a certified instructor. The commitment of attending a class can encourage consistency.

11. Listen to Your Body:

Pay attention to your body and avoid pushing yourself too hard. If you're fatigued or feel pain, it's okay to take a rest day.

12. Track Your Progress:

Keep a journal to record your workouts and progress. Seeing improvements over time can be highly motivating.

13. Stay Informed:

Stay up-to-date with new Wall Pilates techniques and exercises. Learning and trying something new can reignite your enthusiasm.

14. Reward Yourself:

Celebrate your achievements, whether it's mastering a new exercise, reaching a specific goal, or staying consistent for a set period. Treat yourself to a small reward as a motivator.

15. Make It a Habit:

Consistency becomes easier when Wall Pilates becomes a habit. The more regularly you practice, the more natural it becomes.

16. Be Patient:

Understand that progress in Wall Pilates, like any fitness discipline, takes time. Be patient and persistent, and don't be discouraged by temporary plateaus.

17. Get Adequate Rest:

Rest and recovery are crucial. Ensure you get enough sleep and allow your body to recuperate between sessions.

18. Consult with a Professional:

If you encounter challenges or feel unsure about your practice, seek guidance from a certified Wall Pilates instructor or fitness professional.

Maintaining a consistent Wall Pilates practice can lead to improved core strength, flexibility, posture, and overall well-being. By incorporating these strategies into your routine and staying dedicated to your practice, you'll experience the many benefits that Wall Pilates has to offer.

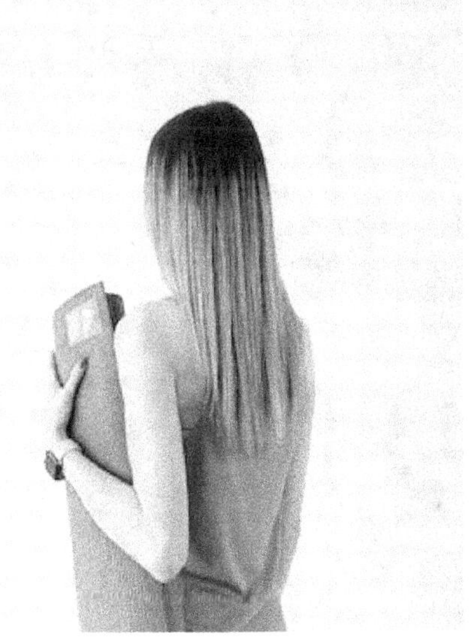

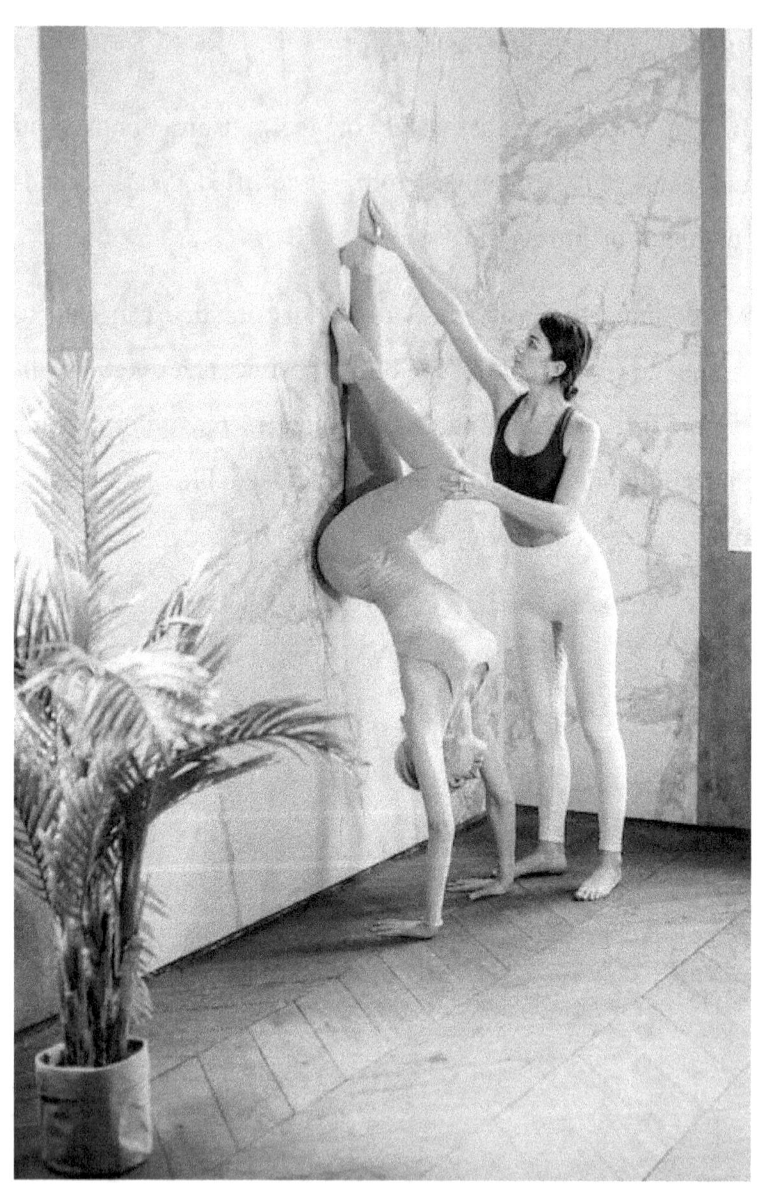

CONCLUSION

In conclusion, Wall Pilates for beginners offers a remarkable journey toward improved fitness, strength, flexibility, and overall well-being. This fusion of classical Pilates principles with the support of a wall provides a safe and effective way for individuals at all fitness levels to embark on a path of holistic self-improvement.

As beginners, you've taken the first crucial step toward enhancing your health and wellness. By focusing on core engagement, precise movements, and controlled breathing, Wall Pilates cultivates a strong mind-body connection.

This practice not only strengthens your muscles but also enhances your posture and flexibility, making everyday activities feel more effortless and enjoyable.

Throughout this guide, you've been introduced to the fundamental exercises, the benefits of Wall Pilates, and the safety precautions that ensure your practice remains injury-free. You've also explored the concept of progression, allowing you to advance at your own pace and challenge your limits.

Your journey as a beginner in Wall Pilates is just the beginning, and the possibilities are endless. As you continue to practice and grow, remember to set clear goals, track your progress, and maintain consistency. Wall Pilates is more than just a workout; it's a way to connect with your body, empower yourself, and experience a profound sense of well-being.

Whether you're seeking a gentle introduction to fitness or a foundation for a more rigorous exercise routine, Wall Pilates for beginners provides a nurturing and transformative experience.

The wall is your steadfast companion, offering support as you explore the art of movement. So, take a deep breath, stand tall, and embrace the journey of Wall Pilates with enthusiasm and dedication.

The benefits you'll reap extend far beyond the physical, touching every facet of your life. Embrace this practice, and witness the positive impact it can have on your health, your body, and your sense of self. Your journey has begun, and the possibilities are boundless.

www.ingramcontent.com/pod-product-compliance
Lightning Source LLC
Chambersburg PA
CBHW070825260726
48660CB00005B/1996